HEALTHY LIVING FOR LONGEVITY:

Learn The Key Practices To Achieving Longevity And Healthy Aging

STEPHEN C. JAMES

Table of Contents

Dedication

When examining the longevity sector, it is evident that far too many individuals are walking down the rabbit holes and becoming lost in the woods. People are hunting for medicinal supplements, utilizing coffee enemas (please don't) and experimenting with intense meditations that have yet to be shown to enhance the human lifespan. Besides, some of the same persons who take these medicines do so after sitting all day and taking down two hamburgers for lunch.

Pursuing a longer healthspan, the duration of time that you're cognitively intact and physically competent does not need to be complex. I dedicate this book to individuals interested in achieving the absolute best for their health, can see beyond the noise, and are searching for a reference to assist you reach your goals.

Introduction

Tales of immortality and endless youth have been handed down between generations for thousands of years. From ancient Greek mythology to current literature and movies, the ideal of living forever has been chronicled extensively across history. While the Fountain of Youth may still only exist in myths and tales, the potential of living longer has become a reality, owing to developments in science, medicine, and public health. But unlike in the myths, the secret to longevity isn't a miraculous potion – it's good behaviors.

Some study predicts that heredity accounts for 25 percent of the variety of an individual's lifetime, while environment and lifestyle variables may influence the remainder. With comparable healthy practices, such as avoiding smoking and keeping a decent weight, people who have lived longest — into their nineties and hundreds — have been found less likely to acquire age-related chronic illnesses, such as heart disease, cancer, and diabetes.

While growing older is inevitable, implementing healthy lifestyle adjustments now may help you age properly, and perhaps add a few additional years to your life.

In this book, you'll learn the evidence-based strategies I have stressed that have been demonstrated to enhance your metabolic health, lower the odds of you suffering from various chronic illnesses and early death, and therefore-in extend your lifetime. So join me on this path towards obtaining maximum metabolic health and longevity.

Chapter 1

Longevity Goals And Why They Are Crucial, Whatever Your Age –What You Should Know About Longevity

If you are fortunate enough to live longer than the usual individual, you may be classified as possessing longevity. Longevity is a mix of health and lifespan that is governed by a multitude of variables.

How to live longer is the age-old topic that is propelling the rapidly-growing longevity ecosystem, which combines research, development, and investment to create longevity solutions. As birth rates decrease and the elderly population continues to expand internationally, human beings' unending search for longer and better lives has never been more vital - but what affects longevity, and how can this be harnessed to help people live longer?

What is Longevity?

Life longevity includes an interaction between healthspan and lifespan, defined as the number of years a person lives in good health and the length of time between birth and death. Life expectancy may drastically vary based on place, for example, the life expectancy in Japan is 81 years contrasted with barely 69 years in Swaziland. According to the Centers for Disease Control and Prevention, the average life expectancy in the United States is 78.8 years.

Individuals' life expectancies are affected by a variety of numerous variables including sex, genetics, lifestyle, and socioeconomic situation. In the US, women on average live around 5 years longer than males, presumably connected to the fact that they are typically less prone to incur risks. Average life expectancy has been growing in the previous several decades from approximately 30-40 years to over 80 years due to changes in food, medicine, and public health.

Longevity tends to be focused in locations known as *'Blue Zones'*, where residents live longer than average everywhere else on earth and where it is normal to observe nonagenarians maintaining active, healthy lives.

Blue Zones exist around the globe across varied cultural landscapes and include the Greek island Ikaria, Okinawa in Japan, and Sardinia in Italy to mention a few. Whether human beings have a maximum lifetime is not entirely known, although some scientists set maximum lifespan estimates at between 120-150 years, this top limit has not yet been achieved.

Healthspan is also crucial to longevity since most individuals never achieve the ideal life as they succumb to age-related sickness. Since no one wants to live for a protracted period of bad health, known as Disability-Adjusted Life-Years (DALYs), this book instead focuses on boosting healthy life expectancy.

Our health is governed by the same mix of genetic and environmental variables that influence longevity. As we age, health steadily degrades and our tendency for acquiring and dying from age-related illnesses including diabetes, cardiovascular disease, and cancer grows.

Aging is an inescapable process that is produced by an accumulation of molecular and cellular damage in the body over time, known as the *'hallmarks of aging'* The chief causes of this damage include genomic instability, attrition of the telomere endcaps of chromosomes, alterations in our epigenetics, and loss of protein homeostasis or *'proteostasis'*.

Therefore, by treating health issues and decreasing the process of aging, life length may be enhanced.

Factors That Impact Longevity

Understanding what drives lifespan is crucial since this information may be used for life-extending therapies. The pace at which we age is governed by a complex mix of lifestyle, genetics, and environment, with the two most significant elements being genes and environment.

Genetics are difficult to control; if one or both parents have a history of heart disease or cancer before the age of 50, there is an increased likelihood that their kids may acquire it too. Equally, life expectancy is to some part impacted by the age at which an individual's parents died.

The environment is also significant to health and longevity; a greater socioeconomic position is related to better health outcomes and life expectancy. This enhances the possibility of access to healthcare, better nutrition, and healthy living surroundings like green areas and clean air.

Living in greater proximity to pollution, as well as ambient air pollution in congested places may induce chronic health concerns. Some of these variables are out of our control, yet there are some actions we can take to lead a better life and boost the chances of an extended lifespan.

Lifestyle changes are the simplest method to keep some control over longevity; for example, smoking, drinking excessive quantities of alcohol, physical inactivity, and eating a bad diet all adversely influence lifespan, but their effect may be lessened with the cessation of these harmful behaviors.

Understanding what drives lifespan is crucial since this information may be used for life-extending therapies.

Improving Healthspan and Lifespan

Life is fundamentally limited, although professionals in the longevity sector have attempted to challenge this by merging advancements in life science and health care with business to disrupt aging and increase health and lifespan.

Since there is no sense in living forever while you are in a permanent state of ill-health, you should instead concentrate on enhancing holistic health and reducing aging, in the hope that this leads to better longevity.

Considering the pace at which human life has expanded over prior centuries, it may likely be prolonged further. Understanding how humans age may be utilized to adopt real-world treatments such as adequate diet, regular exercise, and sleep, as well as AI and diagnostics to enhance health, aging, and overall life longevity.

Chapter 2

Metabolic Health Is Essential To A Longer Healthspan

What is Metabolic Health, and Why is it Important?

You may have noticed various diet strategies over the internet suggesting you improve your metabolism with particular meals and regularly lose weight. This metabolism that they are referring to is the life-sustaining capacity of your body to absorb nutrients and energy from digested food. This procedure serves the objective of beginning development and numerous physiological processes. When your metabolic processes are in flow, there is minimal possibility of acquiring disorders that can harm your general health.

This chapter would assist you to comprehend the definition of metabolic health and advise you on indicators of a not-so-excellent metabolism. You will also discover how you might enhance your metabolic health and profit from it.

Metabolic Health; An Introduction

A healthy metabolism guarantees that your body consumes your meals without adversely influencing your sugar levels, cholesterol, insulin, and inflammation. In addition, it keeps you from acquiring lifelong illnesses that might affect your body's functioning and interaction with food.

Metabolic health is simply defined, as the absence of metabolic disorders. A correctly functioning metabolic health safeguards you from health difficulties including excessive blood sugar, high blood pressure, obesity, fatty liver, renal troubles, cholesterol, etc.

Several things impact your metabolic health. Some of these include heredity, age group, sex, eating habits, physical activity, sleep quality, behaviors like alcohol intake or smoking, stress, and mental health difficulties. There is no set way to boost your metabolic health since each one's metabolic health is unique to them. However, there are specific things you might do to fit your physique.

Importance of Metabolic Health

Your metabolic health is of vital significance to help you maintain a sustainable existence. It safeguards you from the danger of metabolic illnesses and enhances your quality of life.

Metabolic disorders are illnesses that damage the body's capacity to metabolize particular substances or enzymes. In addition, the function of the cell to perform critical biochemical events including the creation of proteins, carbohydrates, and lipids is also impacted by metabolic diseases.

Metabolic health is like what a shell is to a tortoise. The shell protects the tortoise from its predators, similarly, your metabolic health protects you from metabolic problems like diabetes. Therefore, a correct diet and care are important to maintain shell development and health.

Similarly, monitoring your metabolic patterns, consuming the food that helps you, and customized physical exercise to suit you would all contribute to correctly controlled metabolic health. But, again, as you can see out here, personalization is the key.

Can Metabolic Syndrome Define Metabolic Health?

Metabolic syndrome and metabolic health have a direct association. A metabolic syndrome is a group of illnesses that elevate the risk of cardiovascular diseases and other maladies. It is more frequent in adults over the age of 50 years. However, with stress and irregular lifestyles becoming the norm of the day, metabolic syndrome is no longer restricted to elderly persons.

It is generally related to any past family history. It might endure from a few years to a lifetime. Its therapy needs regular monitoring and frequent pathological examinations. Unfortunately, there may be no total treatment yet, however controlling such problems is very much achievable.

Most indicators of metabolic syndrome are typically not taken seriously. Some of them include:

- Increased glucose level, additional signs of diabetes, or borderline diabetes.
- High blood pressure
- High levels of triglyceride and harmful cholesterol
- Being overweight or obese
- Enlargement of waistline

The symptoms of metabolic syndrome in itself will affect metabolic functioning and leave your body sensitive to metabolic disorders including diabetes, mitochondrial dysfunction, and Gaucher's disease, to mention a few. All in all, this would put your metabolic health haywire.

Health Effects

It is normal for your glucose levels, blood pressure, and fat content to increase after having a meal to complete digestion and absorption. However, collecting these increases for a long period is not good. Since everybody's metabolism is distinct, it may go wild in diverse and particular ways. Others people's bodies may create an overabundance of glucose, while some might have excessive blood fat. None of which should be a frequent occurrence.

Consequences of Poor Metabolic Health

The first and greatest indicator of poor metabolic health is unhealthy body weight. It demonstrates that the food intake is higher than what the body can burn. It may suggest the reason as erratic eating and lifestyle choices. Obesity is a worldwide issue. At the foundation of this lies poor metabolic health.

You may develop severe blood sugar, blood pressure, PCOS, and some cancer. Furthermore, evidence shows poor metabolic health might be a factor in diabetes.

You might encounter dietary inflammation, which comes along with oxidative stress. Therefore; weight reduction becomes a byproduct of increased health. The weight immediately begins changing when your metabolic health improves with the correct nutrition and activity measures.

Metabolic cardiology is a relatively emerging discipline of medicine that focuses on preventing, treating, and managing cardiovascular disorders. All of this is taken care of at the cellular level via metabolic interventions that are naturally occurring in the human body.

Improving Your Metabolic Health

Maintaining your metabolic health will demand you to know your health indicators fully and consistently. For example, it entails evaluating your glucose level, weight, body mass, and fat content. Technology helps monitor your health metrics and offers you a place to talk with your health coach and trainer.

Ways To Improve Your Metabolic Health

Knowing your metabolic health may help you find out where you need to make improvements. An RMR test will offer you the information to supply your body with what it needs exactly.

Cutting down on refined sugar, processed and packaged meals, and preserved food products might assist to stabilise excessive glucose variations. Instead, ingest enough fiber-rich plant-based items including seeds, veggies, and whole grains. In addition, drink adequate water and drinks, and eat enough protein, healthy fats, and fiber.

Avoid missing meals, eating fad diets, or keeping an empty stomach for extended hours. It would make you have unnecessary desires and throw your glucose levels out of balance.

You might consume foods high in probiotics or gut microorganisms like yogurt for optimal gut health and assist with dietary inflammation. You could discuss this with your diet coach keeping in mind other parameters.

Exercise or any sort of physical activity for around 30 minutes a day would help you manage your weight and prevent increases in your waistline. Strength training may assist. It would assist in balancing blood glucose and blood pressure and keep your heart healthy. If you have a particular ailment or certain objectives in your mind, you might speak about them to your fitness trainer and tailor the training plan.

A lack of sleep or excess sleep is hazardous to your blood glucose levels. Having a sleep pattern that is not regular might mess with your sugar and produce issues in metabolic working. Make sure you obtain at least 7 hours of night sleep. Research reveals that sleep disturbance, which includes short, poor-quality, and inconsistent sleep, elevates the risk of metabolic problems, including obesity and type 2 diabetes.

Conclusion

A deteriorating metabolism doesn't have to be the inevitable result of age. Managing your health via food, exercise, and ongoing physical and cognitive engagement may promote healthy and effective metabolic aging. A healthy metabolism is a key to a long, wealthy life. And happily, it's largely within your control.

Chapter 3

The Power Of Sleep And Its Impact On Our Longevity

Recent breakthroughs in technology and revolutionary discoveries in science have thrown light on one of the key – but elusive – lifetime aim for many individuals: to live healthier longer lives. The tremendous gain in worldwide life expectancy was among the greatest accomplishments of the 20th century. In 1900, the life expectancy at birth was 31 years — by 2022, it had climbed to approximately 73.

Today, helping individuals age properly is a new healthcare goal. Delaying or even reversing the aging process will have cascading effects on illness prevention and quality of life. Rather than finding a miraculous drug, scientists have begun to explore habits that might be harnessed to boost future generations' life expectancy far above 100 — and they may have a solution.

How about the one habit we perform every single night that already eats up a third of our lives: sleep? This shouldn't come as a surprise. Sleep includes a variety of critical physiological roles including (certainly not limited to):

- Immunity
- Metabolic functioning
- Endocrine (hormonal) functioning
- Cognition
- Thermoregulation
- Waste clearance in the brain

Scientists now think that adequate, regular, and quality sleep may be vital to unlocking a rise in global life expectancy. Research suggests that those persons able to effectively reach extreme old age — the uncommon centenarians who survive to 100

– often have optimum sleep over their lifetime. On the other side, insufficient sleep may hasten the aging process; sleep deprivation impacts practically every physiological function in the body. As a consequence, some research even shows that there is a link between poor sleep and life expectancy.

Sleep Across The Lifespan

Before we go into statistics exploring the association between sleep and longevity, it's crucial to first understand how sleep varies across the lifetime.

As we age, our sleep deteriorates. In reality, sleep substantially alters during a lifetime. So much so, that the amount and quality of our sleep may be utilized as an aperture through which we can examine the brain's aging. Young people tend to have a regular and systematic quantity of sleep phases throughout the night. The night starts with lots of deep sleep, followed by an increase in REM sleep (when we're most likely to dream) throughout the second part of the night.

In elderly persons, this rhythm gets interrupted, and total sleep becomes highly fragmented. The amount of time spent in deep and REM sleep is decreased, and the amount of time spent awake during the night rises.

And it's not simply the amount, or the time spent in these sleep phases, that gets altered. It's the quality of sleep phases that gets affected. The slow waves observed in deep sleep that are essential for many key processes are less strong and less dense as we age. Sleep spindles — a characteristic of NREM sleep — slow down and are less abundant in the elderly. In brief, the brain's capacity to create healthy electrical sleep-related activity reduces as we age.

But this isn't a regular procedure. Older folks don't suddenly need less sleep than they used to — they're just unable to create that *'still'* crucial slumber. There are similarities here with how scientists are starting to think about aging. Some scientists feel it's time to designate aging as a sickness that we should aim to treat, rather than as a natural consequence of life.

Sleep and Longevity

Generally, the study on short sleep duration and lifespan is well characterized. For example, recent research indicates an elevated risk of dementia among people sleeping fewer than 6 hours a night throughout midlife. For example, persistent short sleep duration at ages 50, 60, and 70 compared to persistent normal sleep length was also related to a 30 percent elevated dementia risk irrespective of other possibly driving variables. These data imply that low sleep duration in midlife is connected with an increased risk of late-onset dementia.

Both poor sleep quality and short sleep duration are also connected with decreased glucose metabolism or the mechanism that maintains a continual supply of energy to living cells. After 5 nights of barely 4-hours of sleep, glucose metabolism is affected by up to about 50 percent. We also detect comparable consequences for slow-wave sleep deprivation — underlining the relevance of deep sleep for physiological performance. Taken together, sleep loss' influence on glucose metabolism may encourage the development of obesity, diabetes, and other endocrine/hormonal diseases, further lowering quality of life and severely compromising lifespan.

Optimal Sleep Patterns Associated With Longevity

So, what are the best sleep qualities of people who live long? One research investigated sleep habits in *"the oldest of old individuals"* (those between 85-105 years old) relative to younger and older people (60-70 years old). The researchers showed that individuals with longer lifespans maintained rigorous and regular sleep-wake patterns and kept appropriate amounts of slow-wave (deep) sleep, compared with older people.

Another research explored the link between sleep habits and health in families with remarkable lifespans. The researchers observed that centenarians were protected from age-related variables while being more likely to display symptoms of risk sleep patterns (such as oversleeping and napping), indicating that specific genes may be protective against the negative consequences of sleep disturbance.

Finally, Japanese researchers analyzed the sleep patterns and lifestyle practices of individuals living in Ogimi, a hamlet of longevity. Those in the village that the authors noticed were in *"good sleep health"* were more likely to take short naps, less likely to doze off in the middle of the day, and were more likely to exercise frequently.

Sleep is a fundamental cornerstone for health and wellbeing. Optimal sleep may be the single most crucial pillar for resetting and rebuilding our body, whereas insufficient sleep impairs practically every physiological function in the body and is connected with the genesis and progression of the illness. You may begin to harness the power of sleep by following sleep hygiene advice and making it a non-negotiable priority for your general health, wellbeing, and longevity.

Chapter 4

Importance Of Nutrition For Longevity

What you consume plays a crucial effect on how well you age. Getting the appropriate diet can minimize your risk of numerous age-related disorders and assist you to live a fulfilling life for as long as feasible.

Life expectancy is growing internationally, but a longer life — or more longevity — doesn't always guarantee a healthy one.

Research on the study of nutrition and gut health in the world demonstrates that everyone — even identical twins — responds differently to meals.

To age well, it's necessary to eat excellent quality, natural food. But the healthiest nutrients for your body are unique to you.

How What You Consume Impacts Your Health As You Age

Close studies have demonstrated the consequence of eating meals that aren't beneficial for your body.

These bad consequences include changes to the molecules in your blood, feeling hungry more often, and increases in signs of inflammation. When you harm yourself or get sick, inflammation may be a healthy thing that protects you and helps you to heal. But continued amounts of inflammation can be detrimental.

Over time, the negative impacts of consuming foods that aren't good for you can raise your risk of long-term health concerns, such as heart disease and diabetes, and can also contribute to weight gain.

The Gut Microbiome

Your gut plays an essential part in the way your body responds to food. The colony of microorganisms that dwell in your gut is known as your *'gut microbiome'*. A greater diversity of diverse helpful intestinal bacteria is healthy for you.

Research suggests the gut may harbor 15 *"good bugs"* that are related to better health and 15 *"bad bugs"* linked with lower health.

The harmful bugs are related to an increased risk of type 2 diabetes, heart disease, and extra belly fat.

The good news is that you can adjust your gut microbiome through your diet by including items that assist beneficial microorganisms proliferating in your gut.

As you read, you'll learn it's feasible to discover which of the *"good"* and *"bad"* bugs dwell in your gut and what your particular *"gut booster"* meals are that might aid your *"good"* bugs to thrive.

Blood sugar and Blood fat responses

When you eat, your body breaks down carbs into a simple sugar called *'glucose'*, and it breaks down lipids into *'triglycerides'*.

As the name implies, blood sugar, or blood glucose, is the sugar that's present in your blood. After you eat, your blood sugar rises. In the hours that follow, it falls again. Big spikes and drops — or *"crashes"* — in blood sugar are not healthy for your health.

Research has demonstrated that the way our bodies respond to food varies with age, especially among women. Our results reveal that on average, women have bigger post-meal blood sugar rises as they become older.

Blood fat is the phrase for the level of triglycerides in your blood. Generally, it takes 6–8 hours for your body to eliminate lipids from your blood. Blood fat responses differ across individuals and are an excellent sign of your risk of getting heart disease.

If your blood fat levels rise too high or stay high for too long, it might exacerbate inflammation. Over time, this can damage your arteries, increasing your risk of illnesses such as heart disease, and influence your long-term health.

Measuring how the levels of sugar and fat in your blood fluctuate after eating, and how long it takes them to recover to normal levels, can help you understand how your metabolism functions.

You may then use this knowledge to pick foods that maintain your blood sugar and blood fat levels more steady.

Everyone is Different

Everyone's responses to food are diverse. It's crucial to understand these responses since they can have an influence on your health in later life.

When you understand your answers regarding your blood sugar and blood fat reactions to food, as well as the unique makeup of your gut microbiome you can select the greatest foods for your body and your long-term health.

5 Nutrition recommendations for Healthier Aging

Although knowing your specific sensitivities to food is the greatest approach to nutrition, there are some basic rules you may follow to enhance your overall health and lower your risk of age-related disorders.

1. Eat more plants
Plants are strong in fiber, which feeds your gut flora, but it's also vital for a good bowel movement and for avoiding constipation.

Brightly colored plants contain a form of antioxidant called polyphenol. As well as supplying food for your *"good"* gut microbes, polyphenols have been linked to a reduced risk of illnesses including type 2 diabetes, cancer, and heart disease.

Try to *"eat the rainbow"* by mixing and combining different colored plants. You should aim at consuming 20-30 different plant meals each week.

Research has shown that persons who do this have a more diversified (and hence healthier) mix of intestinal bugs than those who consume fewer than 10 different vegetables a week.

Although 20-30 may sound like a lot of plants, remember that it's throughout all 7 days of the week and may include items like nuts and seeds, as well as veggies and spices.

Even if you don't achieve 20-30 plants right immediately, adding more to your diet is important for your health.

2. Eat probiotic and prebiotic foods
Research reveals that aging might negatively damage your gut flora. To aid with this, you

can look after your stomach by ingesting prebiotics and probiotics.

Probiotics are living bacteria, like those that dwell in your gut, and experts believe that they offer health advantages. You can acquire probiotics from fermented foods.

Popular fermented foods include fermented vegetables like kimchi or sauerkraut, dairy products such as kefir, swiss cheeses, and live yogurt, and fermented tea called kombucha.

Prebiotics are a sort of fiber that nourish *"good"* bacteria, so they're vital if you want your *"good"* gut bugs to grow. You can discover prebiotics in foods including onions, garlic, leeks, asparagus, Jerusalem artichokes, and bananas.

You need to eat both probiotics and prebiotics routinely — ideally daily — if you want to see the advantages.

3. Eat healthy fats
Poor quality or saturated fats are related to heart disease. However, your body requires fats to function correctly.

They are an essential source of energy, encourage cell development, assist absorb some nutrients, and create important hormones.

Try to exchange animal fats, including those in processed meats, butter, and cream, with healthier plant sources of fat, such as nuts, seeds, avocados, and extra virgin olive oil.

4. Drink less alcohol
Aging might reduce your body's alcohol tolerance. And consuming too much alcohol can increase your risk of illnesses including high blood pressure, cancer, liver disease, and stroke.

I don't believe in cutting anything out totally, and the Dietary Guidelines for Americans say that alcohol may be consumed in *'moderation'*. Research has indicated that modest doses of red wine may even have some health advantages, potentially enhancing your digestive health, but then again when it comes to customization, you might need to avoid it altogether if need be.

5. Follow a Mediterranean-style diet
The Mediterranean diet is an eating pattern that incorporates numerous plant-based foods such as cereals, fruits, vegetables, nuts, seeds, and healthy fats like extra virgin olive oil.

Red meat, bad fats, and processed meals are eaten *'infrequently'*, while alcohol — mainly red wine — is enjoyed in moderation.

Studies have indicated that the Mediterranean diet is connected with greater health throughout aging and a decreased risk of various age-related disorders.

Drinking modest amounts of red wine as part of the Mediterranean diet may also be useful for lowering heart disease.

Other lifestyle adjustments that aid with aging.
Eating the appropriate diet is vital for good aging.

Conclusion

Getting older is unavoidable, but the appropriate nutrition may help you age healthily, stay active, and enjoy life to its best.

The foods you eat influence your blood sugar and blood fat regulation, as well as the health of your gut microbiome. Over time, negative responses to eating foods that aren't good for your body and drinking alcohol can lead to a buildup of inflammatory changes and can increase your risk of age-related health conditions, whereas eating more plants, and adding fermented foods to improve your gut health, switching to healthy fats, and keeping your alcohol intake at a moderate or absolute-zero level can all help.

Chapter 5

The Relationship Between Sleep And Nutrition — How They Work Together For Longevity

Diet, like sleep, is one of the cornerstones of health and wellbeing. And they're closely related. Although a solid, balanced diet is crucial for overall health, inadequate sleep over time may undermine many of the advantages of a healthy diet. It's one of the reasons doctors feel sleep is the single most effective pillar for resetting and rejuvenating the brain and body. You may even be able to deliberately harness the power of particular meals to promote sleep.

On the other hand, early research reveals that some meals and beverages–and the time of their intake –might potentially wreak havoc on your sleep.

In this chapter, the most current study and information on the link between food, nutrition, and sleep will be disclosed. By knowing how sleep and nutrition are intimately related, you may adjust your diet – both by what and when you eat – to sleep better and live healthier.

The Effects of Specific Food Types on Sleep

It's crucial to remember that a balanced diet with meals not taken too close to night will likely be adequate for sustaining sound sleep and general health for most individuals. However, new (and very early) research reveals that some whole meals may help sleep for certain individuals.

Several studies have indicated that particular tart cherries may increase both sleep duration and sleep quality in certain people. For example, research on individuals ingesting the Jerte Picota cherry – a unique kind native to the Jerte Valley in Spain – demonstrates that middle-aged and older patients exhibited benefits in sleep onset latency (or the time it takes to fall asleep) and total sleep duration. Another research indicated that individuals who ingested Montmorency tart cherry juice reported less time napping during the day, more overall sleep time at night, and improved sleep efficiency (a ratio of time spent in bed to the total time spent sleeping) (a ratio of time spent in bed to the total time spent sleeping). This research also discovered that individuals had considerably higher levels of the melatonin — an essential hormone responsible for circadian rhythm control.

Not a lover of cherries but seeking another fruit that may assist sleep? One research reported that individuals who had 2 kiwifruits 1 hour before bedtime for four weeks exhibited substantially better sleep efficiency and total sleep time.

So, what's so unique about cherries and kiwis and why may they promote sleep? It turns out they're rich in high concentrations of melatonin, serotonin, and other *"phytonutrients"* that are considered to be vital for sleep-wake control. However, substantially more study is required to determine the appropriate "amount" of each fruit and the best time for when they should be ingested to help sleep.

Another possibly surprising item that has lately made the rounds as a sleep aid is... wait for it... oysters! That's correct — one research has revealed that those slimy (glistening?) delicacies served on the half shell may enhance sleep. In this randomized controlled experiment, individuals who ingested oysters high in zinc and astaxanthin-containing krill reported an increase in sleep quality and a decrease in the time needed to fall asleep.

There are also other food categories that, if taken frequently and not too soon to bedtime, may help promote sleep. Recent research of more than 1,000 young people revealed that women who raised their fruit and vegetable diet by 3+ servings exhibited 2-fold greater chances of alleviating insomnia symptoms, a 20 percent boost in sleep quality, and a 4-minute decrease in the time required to fall asleep.

Nonetheless, with so little research and scant data, it's difficult to extrapolate these results outside of the laboratory. These first findings are encouraging nevertheless and support the hypothesis that specific food habits may enhance not just sleep, but also future health and wellbeing. Future studies may assist broadening these early findings and should also look at other prospective foods that are also known to possess significant quantities of sleep-promoting qualities (such as grapes!).

What About Timing?

In general, most experts believe that eating large meals close to night interferes with the body's process of calming down for sleep. As the body struggles to digest the meal, your sleep might be affected. Studies have indicated that having too much-saturated fat and sugar shortly before sleep might lower the amount of time spent in crucial phases of sleep, such as deep sleep. For these reasons, if you feel you must have a snack close to sleep, try to keep it modest.

Another recommendation is to avoid eating anything hot close to nighttime. Ingredients such as spicy sauce and hot peppers might make you feel uncomfortably heated and interfere with your sleep. Very hot meals might create stomach problems also.

How Alcohol Can Disrupt Sleep

If you're having difficulties falling asleep, it might be tempting to grab an alcoholic beverage. Estimates vary, but as many as 20 percent of Americans use alcohol to help them fall asleep quicker. But did you know that even while alcohol might generate that drowsy sensation, it ends up interfering with sleep later in the night? The effects of drinking persist longer than you would believe. For example, it takes roughly 5 hours for the body to clear alcohol after 4-5 drinks. Moderation and timing are the two critical aspects of limiting the sleep-robbing effects of alcohol.

Alcohol: A Potent REM Sleep Suppressor
Drinking alcohol interferes with sleep by disrupting some phases sleep-notably REM sleep (the period of sleep when dreams are most likely to occur) (the stage of sleep where dreams are most likely to occur). Alcohol is one of the most effective REM

sleep inhibitors. After you fall asleep and alcohol's hypnotic effect wears away after the liver metabolizes alcohol, your sleep becomes interrupted, particularly during the second half of the night where REM sleep is more prevalent. For example, you're likely to have lighter sleep and more frequent moments of being awake. Following an evening of drinking, these waking times may entail getting out of bed to use the restroom, causing an even greater interruption of sleep time.

Even little less than two servings a night may drastically disrupt sleep. The authors discovered the following sleep quality changes with different alcohol consumption:

Low consumption: Less than 2 drinks of alcohol affected sleep quality by ~10 percent

Moderate consumption: Two drinks of alcohol reduced sleep quality by ~25 percent

High consumption: Greater than two servings reduced sleep quality by ~40 percent.

Alcohol and Sleep Disorders

Alcohol also raises the incidence of some sleep disorders and exacerbates the symptoms of current sleep disorders. For example, one research indicated that persons who binged more than 2 days/week had 64 percent larger risks of sleeplessness than non-binge drinkers. Similar effects have been seen in young adults. Among those who reported weekly binge drinking, 56 percent had problems remaining asleep, over half reported issues falling asleep, and 62 percent reported concerns with snoring or sleep apnea.

In addition to insomnia, the authors of a recent systematic analysis revealed that greater levels of alcohol intake raised the risk of obstructive sleep apnea by 25 percent.

To sum it up, even though it's a prevalent notion that consuming alcohol helps you sleep peacefully, the fact is that it leads to fragmented sleep, an increased probability of sleep problems, and feeling unrefreshed in the morning. And, if you had a late night, you may wind up getting less sleep than you need and feeling worse in the morning for that reason too. All of these may lead to daytime sleepiness, trouble focusing, and performance issues; therefore drink less alcohol, reach out for healthier food (eating them at the proper time as well) and have better sleep time.

Chapter 6

Exercise, And How It Might Help you — Start Moving More Often!

It is crucial to remain active and keep moving no matter how old you are. Exercise keeps your body and your brain healthy.

How does it do that? And what's the greatest way to fit it into your life?

Well, read on to find out how exciting it'll be to discover that you don't need to undertake difficult activities to remain Healthy.

Why Exercise Matters

It can help you live a longer, healthier life because it can:

- Keep your bones, muscles, and joints healthy
- Make you less likely to develop problems like diabetes, colon cancer, and osteoporosis
- Lower your blood pressure
- Manage stress and enhance your mood
- Ease symptoms of anxiety and sadness
- Lower your risks of heart disease
- Manage chronic illnesses like arthritis or diabetes by aiding with things like stamina, joint swelling, discomfort, and muscular strength
- Help with your balance, so you're less likely to fall and break bones.

How Much Exercise?

As you become older, you may be a little apprehensive about exercising. Maybe you worry you could damage yourself or that you have to join a gym. Or you may not be sure what workouts you should undertake.

The trick isn't how or where you become active, it's simply to start moving.

While keeping healthy, you should strive for 150 minutes of movement that gets your heart pounding and your blood flowing per week. Sure, you can do it in workout courses. But you may also obtain it via vigorous walking. It's also crucial to execute motions that train all your main muscles at least 2 days a week. Also, attempt to practice flexibility exercises 2 or 3 days a week to aid with your range of motion.

While 150 minutes may seem like a lot, you don't have to do it in huge chunks. You may take a 10-minute stroll around the block or spend 10 minutes sweeping the porch. It all adds up.

If you're feeling energetic (this might apply to elderly athletes), you'll obtain even more health advantages if you work up to 300 minutes or more of exercise a week.

But a simple objective is to attempt to obtain 30 minutes of moderate-intensity activity on most days. You may be able to do it some weeks and not others. Remember, it's a goal and not a rule. Do what works for you.

How to Get Moving

There are two ways to move: exercise and physical activity.

Exercise is an organized activity like aerobics classes, tai chi, spin courses, or swimming. Physical activity is the method you *"sneak"* movement into your day, like walking the dog or gardening. Adding both to your regimen can help you remain healthy and live longer. But always consult with your doctor before suddenly getting more active.

You don't need fancy clothes or equipment. To get in motion in a less formal way, you can:

- Take a fast stroll or jog
- Ride a bike
- Rake leaves, or drive a lawn mower
- Sweep or dust
- Play tennis
- Walk up and down stairs
- Carry groceries

You should start to feel stronger and have more energy in only a few weeks. Then if you feel you're up to it, you may go to the gym or community center and attend water aerobics or dancing courses, or strength-training activities.

The basic objective is to stay moving more frequently than normal; striving to achieve 30 minutes of moderate-intensity exercise on most days. You may be able to accomplish it some days and not others, likewise some weeks and not others. Remember, it's a goal and not a rule. Do what works for you, but don't sit all day!

Chapter 7

The Key Truths For Living Longer And Healthier

Here are the summarized key practices you may apply to live longer and age healthier;

1. Get moving
It's no surprise that exercise is excellent for the body. But in addition to keeping you healthy and strong, frequent physical activity — even in tiny quantities — may also lengthen your longevity. Exercise has been found to lower your risk of age-related illness such as cardiovascular disease, diabetes, stroke, and some cancers, while strengthening your bones and muscles, and enhancing your overall life expectancy. Meanwhile, studies have connected sedentary lifestyles and lack of exercise with an increased risk of early mortality. The

CDC suggests a minimum of 150 minutes of moderate activity per week, but you'll still enjoy the advantages of exercise in lower quantities. One research indicated that simply 15 minutes of physical exercise a day may enhance your longevity by 3 years. Research has also revealed that exercise may reduce and reverse aging on a cellular level.

2. Stop smoking

Smoking is the biggest cause of avoidable mortality in the United States and has been related to illness in virtually every organ of the body. On average, smokers die approximately 10 years sooner than non-smokers and have three times the mortality rate. That being said, it's never too late to stop. Quitting smoking may add as much as 10 years to your life, and minimize the chance of sickness or death from heart attack, heart disease, stroke, lung cancer, and several other cancers. And the younger you stop, the better! Quitting before 40 has been proven to minimize the risk of mortality from smoking-related illness by roughly 90 percent.

3. Drink in moderation

Excessive alcohol consumption can increase your risk of heart disease, liver disease, high blood pressure, and certain cancers — all of which can lead to a shorter life span. According to one study, adults who drink 14 to 25 drinks per week could be shortening their life expectancy by one to two years, while those who drink more than 25 drinks may be shortening their lifespan by four to five years. If you do drink, moderation — one drink per day for women and up to 2 drinks per day for males — is crucial to reducing these harmful health implications. Some studies shows that light to moderate drinking (wine particularly) may even lessen your risk of heart disease or stroke. As personalization comes into play, there's a study demonstrating that even moderate alcohol consumption might be detrimental, therefore there is no need to start drinking if you don't already.

4. Reduce stress

While stress is an inescapable aspect of life, heightened anxiety and worry may take a considerable toll on the body and affect practically all of its systems. Research shows that persistent stress may raise risk of depression, anxiety disorders, heart disease, high blood pressure, diabetes, inflammation, and obesity, as well as reduce life expectancy. According to one Finnish research, for instance, high stress shortened the lifespans of both men and women by nearly 2 years. Luckily, there are various techniques to handle stress and safeguard your mental health, from journaling and yoga, to counseling and meditation.

5. Stay connected

Friendships and relationships are more than simply emotionally rewarding; they are excellent for your physical health too! A clinical assessment of almost 150 research indicated that those with strong social networks, on average, had a 50 percent better probability of surviving than those with less social support. In fact, according to the research, the health risk of social isolation is similar to smoking 15 cigarettes a day and is more important than being fat or sedentary. Having strong, meaningful connections may raise emotions of happiness and general contentment with life, as well as lower stress and improve overall health. Even being supportive of others may be excellent for your health, so make sure to prioritize time for friends and loved ones.

6. Get adequate sleep
A regular sleep pattern is also vital to your body's general functioning. Numerous studies have shown that poor sleep is associated with major health concerns like hypertension, inflammation, diabetes, cardiovascular disease, and obesity – all of

which lead to a shortened lifespan. On the other hand, too much sleep may also be hazardous for your health, since it has been related with a larger risk of stroke and heart disease. To extend your lifespan, strive to go to bed at the same time each night, and aim for at least 7 hours of sleep.

7. Follow a healthy diet

Many individuals prefer to think about their diet in terms of their short-term health objectives, such as weight reduction or improved digestion. But what you consume today may have a profound influence on your life in the long run, including its duration. A nutritious diet, rich in fruits, vegetables, fiber, and whole foods, has been demonstrated to be protective against inflammation and chronic illnesses, such as heart disease, diabetes, obesity, hypertension, and some cancers, that cause the majority of early deaths. One research projected that more than 400,000 deaths a year may be averted with nutritional reform.

And even minor modifications in nutrition may do the job; Improving diet by only 20 percent was shown to cut risk of early mortality by 8 to 17 percent . While there is a lot of discussion regarding which foods promote lifespan, it's preferable to concentrate on consuming a range of full, unprocessed foods throughout most meals. In general, it means eating enough vegetables, fruits, whole grains, nuts, and legumes and cutting down on processed sugars as much as possible. Some studies also reveal a correlation between the Mediterranean diet — a strategy focusing on fish, fruits, vegetables, olive oil, whole grains, and legumes — and longevity, as well as decreased risk of heart disease and diabetes.

Chapter 8

How To Boost Your Fitness And Track Your Progress

While simply trying to get yourself involved in proper dieting and laying off the junk food, getting more sleep which could mean more than not staying up too late, and regular exercise; that is trying to keep fit, as well as tracking your progress and keep being healthy, you should know it won't always come easy. You'll need a smart approach to break some of those harmful behaviors.

You should do this:

- Think About It
- Break It Down
- Set Small Goals
- Swap Bad for Good
- Track Your Progress

- Forgive Yourself

Think About It

Knowing you need to alter something typically isn't enough incentive to accomplish it. You may even believe there's a solid reason you do it.

For example, often individuals who smoke feel that smoke breaks are the only times they can step away from their job throughout the day. And dining together is a way to engage with friends and family, so you may go along with the crowd instead of picking healthier choices.

But are they truly good reasons? You may take a break and walk outdoors without smoking. You may enjoy lunch with friends and make smarter dietary choices.

A excellent strategy to start yourself going is to find out what rewards you'll obtain when you modify your habits:

- You'll feel better when you take care of your health.
- Your risks of some illnesses and ailments may go down.
- More movement and healthier meals might help you drop a few pounds and feel more comfortable in your clothing.
- Getting more sleep will offer you greater energy.
- If you smoke, you'll save money, and your clothing, breath, and house won't smell like smoke after you stop.

Break It Down

If the adjustment feels daunting, start with modest actions and objectives. One method to achieve it is a tactic from the business sector called *SWOT:*

Strengths:
- What are you already doing right?
- What talents do you have?
- Are you an excellent chef who can prepare healthy, tasty meals?
- Are you skilled at scheduling, so you can make time to exercise?
- Who will assist you in this? Friends, relatives, co-workers?

Weaknesses:
- What may go in your way?
- Do you put things off so you don't have time to create nutritious meals or go to the gym?
- Do you have a hard time sleeping due to stress?

Opportunities:
- What could assist you stop your bad habit?
- Can you join a club or support group?
- Does your business have a gym?
- Are there applications that assist you organize your exercises or measure your progress?

Threats:
- Could something you can't control throw a wrench into your plans?
- Does your job schedule regularly change?
- Do those around you attempt to push you to cling to your poor habits?

Plan how you'll react to these problems. Take a minute and put your replies down to assist you navigate through it all.

Set Small Goals

Going cold turkey might be challenging, so start small:

- Instead of avoiding eating sweets, take one less snack each day.
- If you want to be more active, take a brief stroll after supper each night.
- If you can't sleep, set an alarm to remind you to switch off the TV, phone, or computer one hour before you want to go to bed.
- Aim for stuff you're quite confident you can accomplish. Small victories may keep you going.

Swap Bad for Good

It's crucial to replace poor habits with positive ones. Otherwise, you're likely to slide back into your previous patterns.

For example, individuals who stop smoking may replace it with munching. Having healthy alternatives nearby, like fruit, may help prevent that from becoming an issue.

If you switch off the computer in time to wind down and go asleep, but replace it with your phone or the TV, that's probably not going to help. (Light from a screen might keep you awake.) Instead, try meditating, writing in a diary, or reading a book.

A few further tips:

Pick a new healthy habit you like. If you despise jogging on a treadmill, odds are you won't stay with it. If you don't like broccoli, there's no purpose in heaping your plate with it.

Change one habit at a time. Trying to accomplish too much at once might make it so hard to know where to start that you don't start at all. As you accomplish each objective, add another one.

Don't Hurry

Chances are, you didn't create the bad habit overnight, so allow yourself the time to build the new one. It might take 2 to 3 months for a new routine to take hold.

Track Your Progress

Keep a daily note of the adjustments you make. If you haven't accomplished your objectives for the week, think about what went wrong, then see what you may do better next week.

If you've fulfilled your objectives, give yourself a small treat. Seeing things build up, like your exercises or the days since you've had a cigarette, may inspire and encourage you.

Forgive Yourself

Setbacks are typical. Don't beat yourself up when you have one. Think back to when you first started, look at your daily record, and remind yourself of how far you've come. One slip-up doesn't wipe all that away. Then take up where you left off.

Your Longevity Is in Your Hands

Wellness Warriors, if you link aging with inactivity or being *"over the hill"*, you're less inclined to take care of yourself. You'll give in to decline. If you think that aging is determined by how you feel, you're more inclined to pursue good behaviors, establishing a better life span. You'll consume meals that fuel rather than hurt your body. You'll receive the restful sleep you need, so you have the vigor to energize yourself throughout the day. You'll move more and sit less.

All these behaviors will make you feel better—and younger—and, in turn, help you enjoy the greatest possible health for the rest of your life.

Until next time, Live Well, Live Long!